Introduction: Why You Should Work Out

If you're reading this, you've probably heard it a thousand times: "You should work out." But here's the thing—working out is not just a suggestion or a piece of trendy lifestyle advice. It's a necessity. It's the single most effective tool you have to improve every aspect of your life, from your physical health to your mental well-being, emotional stability, and even your spiritual growth. The truth is, working out isn't just about losing weight, building muscle, or looking better in the mirror. Those are great side effects, sure, but they only scratch the surface of what's at stake.

Working out is about strength—not just physical strength, but strength in every sense of the word. It's

about becoming stronger mentally, emotionally, and spiritually.

So why should you work out? Because the alternative is weakness. And weakness has never been a virtue. You owe it to yourself—and everyone else in your life—to be strong, capable, and useful. That starts with working out.

When you choose to work out, you're choosing to invest in yourself, to develop resilience, discipline, and the ability to push through adversity. You're choosing to take control of your health, your mindset, and ultimately, your life.

Physical Health: The Foundation of Well-Being

Your body is your vehicle through life, and if it breaks down, everything else comes to a halt. Regular exercise keeps that vehicle running smoothly. It strengthens your muscles, bones, and joints, improves cardiovascular health, and boosts your metabolism. It reduces the risk of chronic diseases like heart disease, diabetes, and even certain cancers. You age better, with fewer aches and pains, more mobility, and greater independence. When you work out, you're investing in your long-term health, ensuring that as you age, you maintain not just your lifespan but your quality of life. But working out isn't just about living longer; it's about living better. When your body is strong and healthy, everything feels easier. You have more energy, sleep better, and recover faster. Your body becomes an asset, not a liability. Physical health is the foundation for everything else you do, and regular exercise is how you build and maintain that foundation.

Mental and Emotional Health: A Clearer, Stronger Mind

The benefits of working out don't stop at your muscles—they extend to your mind. Exercise is one of the most powerful tools for improving mental health.

When you work out, your brain releases endorphins, serotonin, and dopamine - neurochemicals that reduce stress, lift your mood, and fight off anxiety and depression. It's no coincidence that some of the most mentally resilient people are also the ones who make fitness a regular part of their routine.

Physical activity improves your focus, sharpens your memory, and helps you think more clearly. Regular exercise teaches you discipline, patience, and how to set and achieve goals. These qualities build mental toughness—the ability to push through challenges not just in the gym but in life. When you work out, you train your mind to handle stress, adapt to change, and bounce back from setbacks. The strength you build physically becomes the mental resilience you need to tackle life's challenges.

Emotional Stability: Managing Stress and Building Resilience

Let's face it—life is stressful. Whether it's work, family, relationships, or the daily grind, stress is a constant. Exercise is one of the most effective ways to manage that stress. When you work out, you're not just burning calories—you're burning off tension, frustration, and anxiety. The physical exertion provides a natural emotional release, allowing you to let go of pent-up emotions in a healthy, productive way.

Beyond stress relief, working out helps you build emotional resilience. When you push through a challenging workout, you learn to embrace discomfort and overcome obstacles. That process of pushing through physical limits translates directly into emotional strength. You become more capable of handling life's ups and downs with grace, patience, and a sense of control.

Spiritual Growth: Connection and Purpose

Working out also fosters spiritual well-being. Exercise is a practice in discipline, mindfulness, and presence—qualities that are essential for spiritual growth. Whether it's through the rhythmic breath of running, the quiet focus of yoga, or the mental clarity that comes from a good workout, physical activity connects you to the present moment. It allows you to step outside the noise of daily life and tune into yourself.

For many, working out is a form of moving meditation. It's a time to reflect, reset, and reconnect with a deeper sense of purpose. Through the physical act of working out, you tap into something greater than yourself—the pursuit of self-mastery, growth, and transformation. Exercise becomes a way to honor your body and cultivate a sense of gratitude for your health and well-being.

Why You Can't Afford to Skip It

The benefits of working out are undeniable, and the consequences of neglecting your physical health are equally clear. Without regular exercise, your body weakens, your mental health suffers, and your ability to handle life's challenges diminishes. Over time, the cost of inactivity piles up—aches and pains, low energy, poor mood, and an increased risk of chronic illness. Avoiding exercise is a slow surrender to weakness, illness, and decline.

On the other hand, when you make exercise a priority, you're actively choosing strength, vitality, and resilience. You're not just surviving; you're thriving. You're taking control of your health, your mindset, and your future. No matter where you are starting from, you have the power to change, grow, and improve. Working out is the most direct, effective way to make that happen.

Conclusion: The Choice Is Yours

The choice to work out is a choice to live a better life. It's a commitment to becoming stronger, healthier, and more resilient—not just physically, but mentally, emotionally, and spiritually. Every time you work out, you're investing in your future self. You're building the strength you need to face life's challenges head-on, with confidence and purpose.

So why should you work out? Because the alternative is weakness, stagnation, and decline. Because strength—physical, mental, emotional, and spiritual—is your responsibility. And because you deserve to live the best, fullest, most empowered version of your life. Working out isn't just something you should do—it's something you need to do, for yourself and for the life you want to lead.

It's time to take that step. You have everything to gain and nothing to lose but your limitations.

Chapter 1: The Physical Benefits of Working Out

When most people think of working out, their minds go straight to the physical benefits—and for good reason. Regular exercise improves nearly every system in your body, making you stronger, more resilient, and healthier overall. But the truth is, the full range of benefits extends far beyond looking good in the mirror or hitting a personal best at the gym. Working out profoundly transforms your body, and these changes will serve you throughout your entire life. Let's dive into the major ways physical exercise improves your well-being, making your body not just stronger, but better equipped to handle the demands of everyday life.

Increased Strength and Muscle Mass

The most obvious benefit of working out—especially with resistance training—is increased strength and muscle mass. Muscle is functional tissue; it's not just there for show. It allows you to perform everyday tasks more easily, from carrying groceries to picking up your kids. Every time you lift, push, or pull a weight, you stress your muscles, causing microscopic tears. As your body repairs those tears, the muscles become bigger and stronger. This is the foundation of progressive overload, which means continually challenging your muscles so they adapt and grow. More muscle also means more strength, which makes life easier. When your body is stronger, everything requires less effort. Climbing stairs, lifting objects, or even standing for long periods become more manageable. And as you get older, preserving muscle mass becomes crucial for maintaining independence and preventing falls. Strength is the foundation of all physical health—without it, everything else declines.

Improved Bone Density

Strength training doesn't just build muscle; it strengthens your bones as well. Weight-bearing exercises, whether lifting weights or doing bodyweight movements like push-ups and squats, put stress on your bones. In response, your body builds more bone tissue, increasing bone density. This is particularly important as you age because bone density naturally decreases over time, leading to conditions like osteoporosis.

A stronger skeletal system means you're less likely to suffer fractures or bone-related injuries, especially as you get older. Weight training essentially prepares your bones to withstand the wear and tear of daily life, making them more resilient.

Better Joint Health and Mobility

Exercise improves joint health by strengthening the muscles, tendons, and ligaments that support your joints. A well-rounded workout routine includes a full range of motion, which helps maintain and even improve mobility. The more you use your joints properly, the better they function. Resistance training can also prevent or reduce the risk of joint problems like arthritis.

When you train regularly, particularly with movements that mimic everyday activities (like squats or deadlifts), you improve your body's ability to move freely and efficiently. This means fewer aches and pains, a reduced risk of injury, and the ability to move through life more comfortably.

Enhanced Cardiovascular Health

Though resistance training is often associated with building muscle, it also benefits your cardiovascular system. Strength training increases your heart rate, especially during intense sets. When combined with cardio exercises like running, cycling, or swimming, it creates a powerful effect on your heart and lungs. Regular exercise strengthens the heart, making it more efficient at pumping blood. This lowers your resting heart rate, reduces blood pressure, and improves circulation. A healthier cardiovascular system means a reduced risk of heart disease, stroke, and other cardiovascular conditions. It also means you'll have more endurance for physical activities—whether it's going for a hike, playing sports, or just walking around your neighborhood.

5. Better Body Composition

One of the most noticeable benefits of working out is how it changes your body composition. This isn't just about losing weight or gaining muscle—it's about the ratio of lean mass (muscle) to fat. Strength training helps build muscle, while cardiovascular exercise burns calories and reduces body fat. Together, they create a leaner, more efficient body.

Carrying less fat and more muscle isn't just about aesthetics. Excess body fat, particularly around the abdomen, is linked to an increased risk of various diseases, including heart disease, diabetes, and certain cancers. Improving your body composition by increasing muscle mass and reducing fat can drastically improve your health outcomes in the long term.

Increased Metabolism

One of the often-overlooked benefits of building muscle is its impact on your metabolism. Muscle is metabolically active tissue, meaning it requires more energy to maintain than fat does. The more muscle you have, the more calories you burn throughout the day— even when you're resting.

This is called the "afterburn effect" (excess post-exercise oxygen consumption, or EPOC), which means your body continues to burn calories after a workout as it works to return to its normal state. Strength training is particularly effective at increasing EPOC, which makes it a powerful tool for improving metabolism and helping with fat loss.

Improved Posture and Balance

Working out, especially through strength training and functional movements, significantly improves posture and balance. Poor posture often stems from weak muscles, particularly in the core, back, and hips. By strengthening these areas, you improve your body's alignment and ability to stay upright. This doesn't just make you look better—it also reduces chronic pain, particularly in the lower back and neck.

Better posture and balance also reduce the risk of injury, particularly falls as you age. Strengthening your muscles, joints, and core gives you better control over your movements, making everyday tasks and sudden movements safer.

Enhanced Flexibility

Many forms of exercise, especially strength training with a full range of motion and stretching practices like yoga, improve flexibility. Flexibility allows your muscles and joints to move freely and without pain. This not only prevents injuries but also improves performance in both daily activities and athletic pursuits.

Improved flexibility also reduces stiffness and discomfort, which is especially important as you age. Being able to move through a full range of motion without pain makes life's tasks easier—from bending over to tie your shoes to reaching for something on a high shelf.

Boosted Immune System

Regular exercise can give your immune system a boost. Physical activity improves circulation, allowing immune cells to move through your body more effectively and identify threats like bacteria or viruses. It also helps to reduce chronic inflammation, which weakens your immune defenses.

Additionally, exercise can help flush bacteria out of the lungs and airways, reducing your chance of getting colds or other illnesses. While intense, prolonged exercise can temporarily lower immune function, moderate regular exercise has long-term benefits for immune health.

Longevity and Vitality

Perhaps the most powerful benefit of regular exercise is that it enhances longevity and vitality. Studies consistently show that people who exercise regularly live longer and enjoy a higher quality of life as they age. Working out helps prevent many of the chronic diseases that shorten life expectancy, including heart disease, diabetes, and certain cancers.

Regular exercise also keeps you physically capable as you age, preserving muscle mass, mobility, and independence. Aging is inevitable, but how you age is largely up to you. By committing to regular exercise, you not only extend your lifespan but ensure that the years you add are lived in good health, free from unnecessary physical limitations.

Conclusion

Working out is one of the most powerful tools you have for improving your physical well-being. It builds strength, improves your cardiovascular health, enhances flexibility, and promotes better body composition. But beyond these obvious benefits, exercise prepares your body to thrive in every aspect of life. It makes you more resilient, reduces your risk of injury, and keeps you moving freely for decades to come.

Chapter 2: The Mental and Emotional Benefits of Working Out

We all know that exercise is good for the body, but the impact it has on your mind and emotions can be just as profound. In fact, for many people, the mental and emotional benefits of working out are what keep them coming back, even on days when motivation might be low. The reality is that your mind and body are deeply connected, and when you take care of one, the other naturally benefits as well. Working out is one of the most powerful tools for improving mental health, reducing stress, and building emotional resilience. In this chapter, we'll explore how regular physical activity can enhance your mental clarity, emotional stability, and overall well-being.

Reduces Stress and Anxiety

Life is stressful, and no one is immune to its pressures. Whether it's work, relationships, or the endless demands of daily life, stress can take a toll on your mental health. Exercise is a highly effective way to reduce stress and anxiety. When you work out, your body releases endorphins—often referred to as "feel-good" chemicals—which naturally elevate your mood and reduce feelings of tension. These endorphins interact with the receptors in your brain, reducing your perception of pain and promoting a sense of calm and relaxation.

Beyond the immediate boost, regular physical activity lowers levels of stress hormones like cortisol and adrenaline, helping you manage daily pressures more effectively. When you incorporate exercise into your routine, you're building a natural defense system against stress. It's not that life becomes less stressful, but you become better equipped to handle it.

Boosts Mood and Fights Depression

Exercise is often described as nature's antidepressant, and for good reason. Numerous studies have shown that regular physical activity can help reduce symptoms of depression. In fact, for mild to moderate cases of depression, exercise has been found to be as effective as medication in improving mood. The reason for this lies in how exercise affects your brain chemistry. It stimulates the production of neurotransmitters like serotonin and dopamine, which play key roles in mood regulation, motivation, and feelings of pleasure.

When you exercise, especially through aerobic activities like running, cycling, or swimming, your brain undergoes changes that make you feel better—not just during the workout, but long after. That post-exercise "high" is a real phenomenon, and it's one of the most powerful natural tools we have for improving mental health. For many people, regular exercise provides structure, routine, and a sense of accomplishment, all of which can help combat feelings of hopelessness and despair.

Increases Mental Clarity and Focus

Working out doesn't just improve your body; it sharpens your mind. Physical activity boosts blood flow to the brain, delivering more oxygen and nutrients, which enhances cognitive function. This improved circulation helps with focus, memory, and problem-solving abilities. You've likely noticed that after a workout, you feel more clear-headed and mentally sharp. This isn't just in your imagination—exercise has been shown to improve concentration and cognitive performance, both immediately after a workout and over the long term.

In fact, regular exercise has been linked to neurogenesis, or the creation of new brain cells, particularly in the hippocampus, the part of the brain responsible for learning and memory. This means that by working out regularly, you're not only improving your short-term mental clarity but also protecting your brain against cognitive decline as you age.

Builds Emotional Resilience

One of the greatest emotional benefits of working out is that it builds resilience. Every time you push through a tough workout—whether it's finishing that last set of squats, running an extra mile, or holding a challenging yoga pose—you're training your mind to persevere. This process of confronting and overcoming physical challenges translates directly into emotional strength. When you push past physical discomfort, you build mental toughness, which helps you handle emotional difficulties more effectively.

Working out teaches you how to cope with discomfort, frustration, and setbacks. These lessons carry over into other areas of life. When you face challenges outside of the gym, you've already trained yourself to handle stress, push through adversity, and keep going, even when things get tough. Over time, this builds emotional resilience, making you more capable of bouncing back from life's inevitable ups and downs.

Improves Sleep Quality

Sleep is crucial for mental health, and working out can significantly improve the quality of your sleep. Regular exercise helps regulate your circadian rhythm, making it easier to fall asleep and stay asleep. It also reduces symptoms of insomnia and improves deep sleep, the most restorative phase of the sleep cycle.

When you sleep better, your brain functions better. You wake up feeling refreshed, mentally sharper, and better equipped to handle the day's challenges. Improved sleep quality also has a direct impact on mood and emotional stability. Poor sleep is linked to irritability, anxiety, and even depression, while quality sleep helps you feel more balanced and in control of your emotions.

Boosts Self-Confidence and Self-Esteem

Exercise doesn't just transform your body—it transforms how you see yourself. As you set goals, work toward them, and see progress, your self-confidence naturally improves. Whether it's lifting heavier weights, running longer distances, or simply noticing changes in your body, each accomplishment reinforces a sense of capability and self-worth.

This increased self-confidence doesn't just come from the physical changes you see in the mirror. It's the result of knowing you've worked hard, challenged yourself, and pushed through discomfort to achieve something meaningful. When you regularly commit to exercise, you build a sense of discipline and self-respect, which boosts your overall self-esteem.

Provides a Healthy Emotional Outlet

Life can be overwhelming, and sometimes we need a healthy way to release pent-up emotions. Exercise provides a productive outlet for stress, frustration, anger, and other intense feelings. Whether you're pounding out your frustrations on a treadmill, channeling stress into heavy lifts, or finding peace in the rhythmic flow of yoga, physical activity gives you a safe and effective way to release negative emotions. After a workout, you often feel lighter, calmer, and more at peace. This emotional release can prevent you from bottling up stress or frustration, which, if left unaddressed, can lead to emotional burnout or even physical illness. Working out provides a natural and healthy way to process and release emotions, helping you feel more balanced and in control.

Cultivates Mindfulness and Presence

Certain types of exercise, like yoga, tai chi, or even mindful strength training, emphasize the importance of being present and fully engaged in the moment. These practices combine physical movement with mindful breathing and focus, creating a powerful sense of awareness and presence. This mindfulness not only enhances the effectiveness of your workouts but also spills over into your daily life, helping you feel more grounded and present.

When you learn to tune into your body's movements, breath, and sensations during a workout, you cultivate a sense of mindfulness that can reduce stress, improve emotional regulation, and enhance your overall well-being. The ability to be fully present in the moment—whether during a workout or in life—fosters a sense of inner peace and emotional stability.

Creates a Sense of Accomplishment and Purpose

Setting and achieving fitness goals, whether it's running your first 5K, hitting a personal record in the gym, or simply sticking to a consistent routine, provides a deep sense of accomplishment. This achievement is more than just physical; it gives you a sense of purpose and direction.

When you see the results of your hard work, you experience a boost in self-worth and a feeling that you're capable of accomplishing whatever you set your mind to. This sense of achievement can positively impact other areas of your life, from your career to your relationships, reinforcing a positive cycle of personal growth and emotional well-being.

Acts as a Social Outlet

Many people find that exercising with others—whether in group classes, team sports, or lifting with a partner—can provide a sense of community and support. Social interaction during physical activity reduces feelings of loneliness and isolation, both of which contribute to poor mental health. Positive social engagement, coupled with the natural mood-boosting effects of exercise, can improve your overall sense of well-being.

Conclusion

Working out isn't just about physical strength—it's a powerful tool for improving your mental and emotional health. It reduces stress, boosts mood, sharpens focus, and builds emotional resilience. Regular exercise helps you sleep better, feel more confident, and provides a healthy outlet for processing emotions. Whether you're looking to reduce anxiety, fight off depression, or simply feel more balanced and in control of your life, working out is one of the most effective ways to improve your mental and emotional well-being.

Incorporating regular physical activity into your life isn't just an investment in your body—it's an investment in your mind and spirit. The benefits go far beyond the gym, helping you become mentally stronger, emotionally more stable, and better equipped to handle life's challenges with grace and resilience.

Chapter 3: The Spiritual Benefits of Working Out

When most people think about working out, they focus on the physical and mental benefits. Rarely does the conversation turn to the spiritual side of exercise, but the connection between body, mind, and spirit is undeniable. The pursuit of strength, discipline, and perseverance through physical exercise has a profound impact on your spiritual well-being. Working out, at its core, is a journey of self-discovery and personal growth. It's a practice that brings you closer to understanding yourself, the world around you, and your place within it. In this chapter, we'll explore how working out can elevate your spiritual life and help you cultivate a deeper connection with yourself and the universe.

Cultivating Discipline and Self-Mastery

At the heart of any spiritual practice is the idea of discipline and self-mastery. Whether through prayer, meditation, or following a spiritual path, discipline is essential for deepening your spiritual awareness. Working out shares this same principle. It requires consistent effort, dedication, and the ability to overcome discomfort in pursuit of growth.

Every time you step into the gym, lace up your running shoes, or unroll your yoga mat, you're practicing discipline. This consistent commitment to physical improvement spills over into your spiritual life. It teaches you the value of persistence, patience, and sacrifice—qualities that are essential for spiritual growth. Through the daily practice of pushing your physical limits, you begin to understand that mastery over the body leads to mastery over the self. When you conquer physical challenges, you develop the mental

fortitude and spiritual discipline to overcome emotional
and spiritual challenges as well.

Connecting Body and Mind

The body and mind are often viewed as separate
entities, but working out reveals their deep connection.
Physical exercise can be a meditative practice that
teaches you to be fully present in the moment. Whether
you're lifting weights, running, or practicing yoga,
working out requires you to focus on your body, breath,
and movement. This mindfulness draws you into the
present moment, quieting the chatter of the mind and
fostering a sense of inner peace.

In many spiritual traditions, the body is seen as a
temple or vessel for the spirit. By taking care of your
body through exercise, you're honoring this vessel and
preparing it to support higher levels of consciousness
and awareness. When you move with intention and
mindfulness, exercise becomes a form of moving

meditation, deepening your spiritual connection and helping you align your physical, mental, and spiritual selves.

Embracing Growth and Transformation

Spirituality is, at its core, about growth and transformation. It's about shedding the old, unproductive parts of yourself and evolving into something stronger, more enlightened, and more connected to a greater purpose. Working out mirrors this journey of transformation. Every time you push through a tough workout or strive for a new personal best, you're literally transforming your body, but you're also transforming your spirit.

Exercise teaches you that growth is a process. There are no shortcuts. You have to put in the work, embrace the discomfort, and trust the process. This mindset is crucial for spiritual growth as well. Just as your muscles adapt and grow stronger with time, so does your spirit as you commit to self-improvement and personal evolution.

Developing a Sense of Presence and Mindfulness

Many spiritual practices emphasize the importance of presence—being fully engaged in the here and now. Working out naturally cultivates this sense of presence. When you're lifting heavy weights, sprinting up a hill, or holding a difficult yoga pose, you have no choice but to focus entirely on the task at hand. Your mind and body must work together, fully immersed in the present moment.

This state of mindfulness, or "flow," is deeply connected to spiritual well-being. It allows you to step outside of the constant stream of thoughts, worries, and distractions that often fill your day. By focusing entirely on your body's movements and sensations, you're practicing the kind of presence that many spiritual disciplines aim to develop. This state of flow can bring about feelings of inner peace, clarity, and a deeper connection to yourself and the universe.

Learning Humility and Acceptance

Physical exercise, especially challenging workouts, often brings you face-to-face with your own limitations. Whether it's struggling to complete a set, gasping for breath at the end of a run, or realizing that progress is slower than expected, working out teaches you humility. It reminds you that you are human, with limits and weaknesses. This humility is an essential aspect of spiritual growth.

Working out also teaches you acceptance. Some days, your body will perform well; other days, it won't. You might have setbacks, injuries, or days when you feel weak. Accepting these ups and downs is key to maintaining a healthy relationship with exercise—and with yourself. This acceptance of your physical self mirrors the spiritual practice of embracing life's challenges and recognizing that everything is part of a larger journey. You learn to let go of perfectionism and embrace the process, both in your workouts and in your spiritual life.

Building a Sense of Gratitude

Exercise, when done consistently, fosters a deep sense of gratitude for your body and its capabilities. Each workout is a reminder of the strength, endurance, and resilience your body possesses. Whether you're running, lifting, stretching, or practicing martial arts, you become more attuned to what your body can do, and this awareness cultivates gratitude.

Gratitude is a powerful spiritual tool. When you appreciate your body for its ability to move, grow, and adapt, you develop a deeper sense of reverence for the life force that animates it. You begin to see your body not just as a vehicle for physical strength but as a sacred gift that enables you to experience life fully. This gratitude extends beyond the gym, helping you feel more connected to the present moment and to the world around you.

Finding Inner Peace through Movement

Many people find that working out provides them with a sense of inner peace and emotional release. Physical activity can help you process difficult emotions and relieve stress, clearing the mental clutter that often blocks spiritual clarity. Movement, in all its forms, has been used for centuries as a way to connect with the divine. From the whirling dervishes of Sufism to the mindful movements of Tai Chi, physical activity has long been recognized as a spiritual practice.

When you engage in exercise, you give your mind and body the opportunity to sync up and release any built-up tension or negativity. This release creates space for inner peace and clarity. After a workout, many people experience a sense of calm and serenity that allows for deeper introspection and spiritual connection.

Connecting with Something Greater

There's a sense of transcendence that comes from pushing your body beyond what you thought possible. Whether you're running a marathon, lifting a new personal best, or simply finishing a challenging workout, there's a moment when you tap into a force greater than yourself. You realize that your strength is not just physical; it's connected to something larger. This sense of transcendence can feel spiritual, as though you've tapped into a deeper source of energy, one that goes beyond your individual self.

Many people find that physical challenges—whether it's hiking in nature, completing a difficult workout, or participating in an athletic event—create moments of connection to a higher power, the universe, or a sense of oneness with the world. These moments remind you that you are part of something bigger, that your individual effort is connected to a greater whole.

Conclusion

Working out is far more than just a physical pursuit—it's a spiritual practice that connects the body, mind, and spirit. Through discipline, mindfulness, and self-mastery, exercise becomes a pathway to deeper self-awareness and spiritual growth. The process of physical transformation mirrors the spiritual journey, teaching you to embrace discomfort, accept your limitations, and cultivate gratitude for the present moment.

Whether you're looking to deepen your connection with yourself, find inner peace, or simply explore the relationship between body and spirit, working out offers a powerful avenue for spiritual well-being. Each workout is an opportunity to tap into a deeper sense of presence, purpose, and connection to the world around you. By caring for your body, you're also nurturing your soul, creating harmony between the physical and the spiritual in your daily life.

Conclusion: The Holistic Power of Working Out

By now, it should be clear that working out isn't just about building muscle, losing weight, or running faster—it's about cultivating a stronger, healthier, and more balanced version of yourself. When you commit to regular exercise, the benefits ripple through every part of your life, creating profound changes not only in your physical body but also in your mental, emotional, and spiritual well-being.

Working out is a holistic practice that transcends the limits of the gym or the track. It's about the way you show up in life, how you handle stress, how you connect with yourself and others, and how you pursue growth in every dimension of your being.

You can have all the information in the world, but it's useless unless you apply it. This is where most people fail. They spend more time thinking about getting in shape than actually doing the work. Here's the cold, hard truth: There's no secret formula, no hack, no shortcut that will get you where you want to go without putting in the effort. You must be consistent. You must embrace the process. And you must understand that progress comes slowly, but it comes.

Understand this: Working out is the clearest, most direct way to teach yourself how to face challenges head-on. It's a practice that can't be faked. You either put in the work, or you don't. You can't cheat the iron. You can't shortcut endurance. And that's why it's so valuable. It's a constant reminder that the best things in life—the things that matter—come through effort, persistence, and sacrifice.

Let's bring together what we've learned about how exercise improves your overall well-being:

Physical Well-Being: Strength, Health, and Longevity

At its most obvious level, working out improves your physical health. Through strength training, cardio, and flexibility work, you build stronger muscles, denser bones, and a more resilient cardiovascular system. This doesn't just make you look better; it makes you move better, feel better, and live better. Your body becomes more efficient at handling the physical demands of everyday life, reducing the risk of injury, disease, and the decline that naturally comes with aging.

Regular exercise keeps your body functioning at its best, helping to prevent chronic conditions like heart disease, diabetes, and osteoporosis. It strengthens your joints, increases your energy, and even enhances your immune system. Most importantly, working out improves your longevity and quality of life, allowing you to live not just longer, but with more vitality and independence as you age.

Mental and Emotional Well-Being: Clarity, Resilience, and Peace

Exercise is one of the most effective tools for managing your mental and emotional health. It reduces stress by releasing endorphins, the body's natural mood elevators, and helps lower levels of cortisol, the stress hormone. Whether you're dealing with anxiety, depression, or just the pressures of daily life, working out provides a powerful emotional release and helps stabilize your mood.

Beyond stress relief, exercise improves cognitive function, enhancing focus, memory, and creativity. It fosters mental clarity, allowing you to think more clearly and make better decisions. But perhaps most importantly, regular exercise builds emotional resilience. Each time you push through a tough workout, you're training your mind to handle adversity and discomfort. This mental toughness extends far beyond the gym, helping you face life's challenges with greater confidence and composure.

By improving your mood, boosting your self-esteem, and helping you manage your emotions more effectively, working out becomes a cornerstone of emotional balance and mental well-being.

Spiritual Well-Being: Connection, Purpose, and Presence

Working out is also a profoundly spiritual practice, even if it's not always framed that way. At its core, exercise teaches you about discipline, perseverance, and the pursuit of personal growth—values that are central to spiritual well-being. Each workout is a practice in mindfulness, forcing you to be present with your body and breath, cultivating a sense of peace and connection with yourself.

As you move your body, you tap into a deeper awareness of its capabilities and limitations. This fosters a sense of gratitude, not only for the physical strength you're building but for the life force that animates it. Exercise becomes a way to honor your body as a sacred vessel and to align your physical actions with your spiritual intentions.

The discipline and perseverance you develop in your workouts mirror the qualities needed for spiritual growth. The humility you cultivate when facing physical challenges teaches you to accept life's ups and downs with grace. And the moments of flow and presence you experience during physical activity connect you to something greater than yourself, reminding you that you are part of a larger, interconnected whole.

The Integrated Journey of Well-Being

When you commit to working out, you're not just transforming your body—you're embarking on an integrated journey that strengthens every part of your being. Physical health lays the foundation for mental clarity and emotional balance, which in turn opens the door to deeper spiritual growth. Each dimension of well-being supports the others, creating a cycle of improvement that elevates your entire life.

Your physical strength enhances your mental toughness. Your mental clarity brings greater emotional resilience. And your emotional balance creates the peace and presence necessary for spiritual connection. Working out is the practice that ties it all together, grounding your well-being in action and experience. It's through the physical practice of moving your body that you nurture your mind and spirit, creating harmony between all aspects of yourself.

The Journey Ahead: Lifelong Growth

Working out is not just a temporary fix or a short-term project—it's a lifelong practice of growth and self-improvement. As you continue to challenge your body, mind, and spirit through regular exercise, you'll find that the benefits keep evolving. What starts as a physical transformation soon becomes a mental, emotional, and spiritual one as well.

There will be days when the motivation isn't there, when the challenges seem too great, or when progress feels slow. But these are the moments that matter the most. Every time you push through resistance—whether it's physical, mental, or emotional—you're building resilience, deepening your connection with yourself, and growing stronger in ways you can't always see.

Remember, this journey is not about perfection, but progress. It's about showing up for yourself day after day, knowing that each small effort brings you closer to the person you want to become. The strength you build, both inside and out, will not only improve your quality of life but will also help you navigate the challenges, joys, and opportunities that life presents.

So keep moving. Keep lifting. Keep running, stretching, and growing. Every workout is an opportunity to improve your physical health, sharpen your mind, balance your emotions, and deepen your spiritual connection. In doing so, you become not just a stronger version of yourself, but a more complete, centered, and fulfilled human being.

Your well-being—physical, mental, emotional, and spiritual—is in your hands. And every time you choose to move your body, you're choosing to elevate your entire life. When you finish reading this book and set it down, the responsibility shifts to you. No one else can do the work for you. No one else will lift the weights, run the miles, or grind

through the hard days. But if you commit to the

process, day after day, you'll find that strength isn't

just something you have; it's something you

become.